Pomegranate - The Super Fruit

A Thousand Year Secret Healing Power Revealed!

Learn How to prevent Heart Disease, High Cholesterol, Stroke and So Much More

By

Jasmin Carerra

Published by:

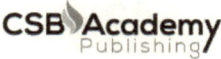

CSB Academy Publishing Company.
P.O. Box 966
Semmes, Alabama 36575

Cover & Interior designed
By
Angie Anderson

First Edition

TABLE OF CONTENTS

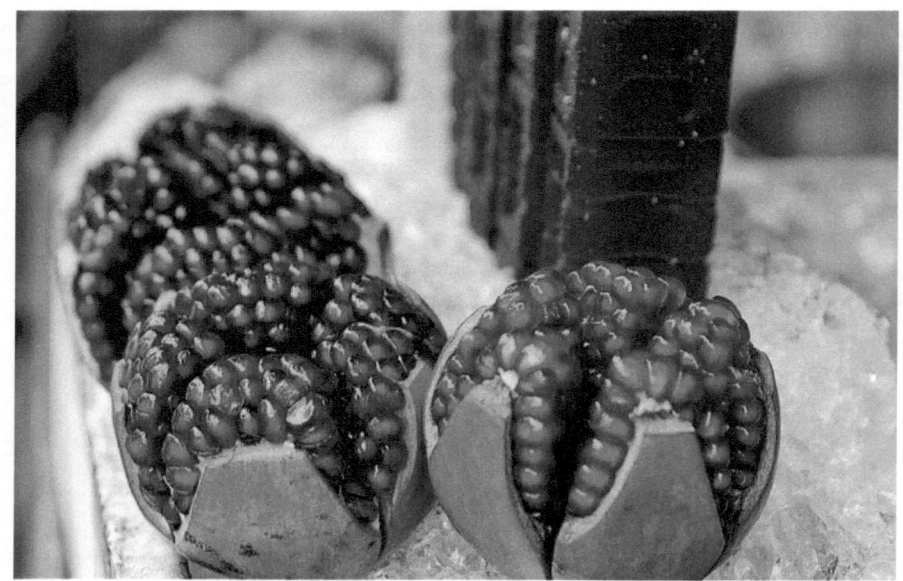

FOREWORD

Each of us probably knows someone who suffers from one or more so-called "diseases of civilization." These diseases - which include obesity, diabetes, hypertension, stroke, high cholesterol and heart disease - are ailments that seem to disproportionately affect members of Western society compared to those in other parts of the world. Oddly enough, all of the diseases mentioned above are affected in some way by your diet.

For years, I lived with extra weight. Okay, "extra weight" is underselling it a bit. I was obese. Not just that, but I suffered from a battery of related illnesses that often go hand-in-hand with obesity, namely high cholesterol, high blood pressure and diabetes. At one point, my doctor warned me that my dietary habits had me on a surefire collision course and if something in me didn't change, no amount of prescription-writing could save me from the fate that lay ahead – heart disease.

Well, you know doctors. They offer lots of advice and plenty of stern warnings. You can get sort of immune. I did. Needless to say, I didn't listen. That is, until a bout with chest pain landed me in the ER. I'd had a heart attack.

That warning I heeded.

I decided the doctor was right. If I was going to live and enjoy a good quality of life, I had to change my habits once and for all. It wasn't easy at first. If you have ever attempted to swap out your old habits for new habits, you probably know what I mean.

Some habits, like eating, require more than just a simple menu change. In order for my changes to be effective long-term, I had to learn what it would take to stay healthy and promote my desire for a better lifestyle over my emotional desire for a temporary sugar-high, which food often provided for me. Not easy, but certainly doable.

The first thing I did was cut back on my intake of refined sugars (love 'em) and simple carbs (doubly love 'em). Talk about painful. The next thing I did was conducted some serious research on alternative medicine and all-natural healing techniques. I studied Ayurveda. Ayurveda is the Hindu system of medicine that focuses on creating and maintaining balance in your body using diet and herbal remedies. I even took a trip to India to really gain some insight into ways to use Ayurvedic medicine to help my body heal from years and years of malnutrition (you can be both fat and malnourished) and dietary abuse. The trip was both eye-opening and, I believe, life-saving.

My research helped me to uncover and successfully apply natural healing techniques to restore my body's natural balance. After a lifetime of developing and solidifying my poor diet habits, it took just a few years for me to unlearn my poor nutrition habits and train my body to long for the foods that would help to keep it disease-free. Believe it or not, a significant part of that discovery centers on the healing qualities of the pomegranate.

My goal is to share what I learned, specifically about the healing power of pomegranate, in this easy-to-read guide. Maybe I can help to keep you from going down the same road I took. And maybe – just maybe – help you to restore your own health.

This book is intended as a reference volume only, not as a medical manual. The information provided in this guide is designed to help you make informed decisions about your health. It is not intended as a substitute for any treatment that may have been prescribed by your doctor. If you suspect you have a medical problem, I strongly urge you to seek competent medical help.

For more information on my findings, please feel free to visit my site www.pomegranatejuicebenefit.com.

PART ONE:

ALL ABOUT THE POMEGRANATE

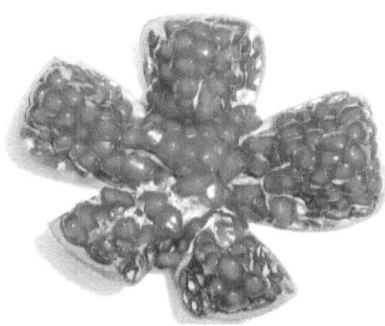

Some call it "the jewel of autumn," and that is quite possibly one of the most descriptive and fitting names for the magical fruit more commonly known as the pomegranate.

For thousands of years, the pomegranate has been a staple in the human diet. Its use dates back to antiquity. Members of the Western World may have only recently discovered the remarkable health benefits of this delicious fruit. But the pomegranate has earned its famed across the globe for its distinctive taste, fetching beauty, and the wide range of health benefits the fruit provides.

The pomegranate is what we call a super food. It is a nutrient-packed, naturally-occurring food that does not have to undergo any sort of processing to be nutritionally valuable. Just pick and eat. Like any super food, the pomegranate delivers a real nutritional punch to any diet. It has documented medicinal benefits. It helps to prevent, control and eliminate some common, everyday ailments. The healing power of the pomegranate is not just the stuff of ancient legend either. Its medicinal properties have been proven through centuries of use in traditional medicine as well as controlled scientific case studies steeped in modern science.

The pomegranate is technically a berry that grows best in warm climates. Pomegranates – the ones we typically see in the grocery stores between October and January – are deep red in color with a thick, leathery skin (or rind) wrapped around the outside of the fruit. Inside, hundreds of small, edible, red arils are separated into bunches by thin layers of white, non-edible membranes. The membranes are not poisonous to eat, but they are rather astringent and don't taste so good. The arils are actually seeds encased in a sweet, juicy pulp covered in thin skin. After carefully removing the outer skin of the fruit and the white membranes, the arils can be enjoyed as a delightful and nutritious treat.

The pomegranate goes by many different names. Perhaps you are familiar with some of these: punic apple, grenade, Indian apple, granatapfel, Chinese apple, granada, seeded apple, melograno, fruit of the dead, and melagrana.

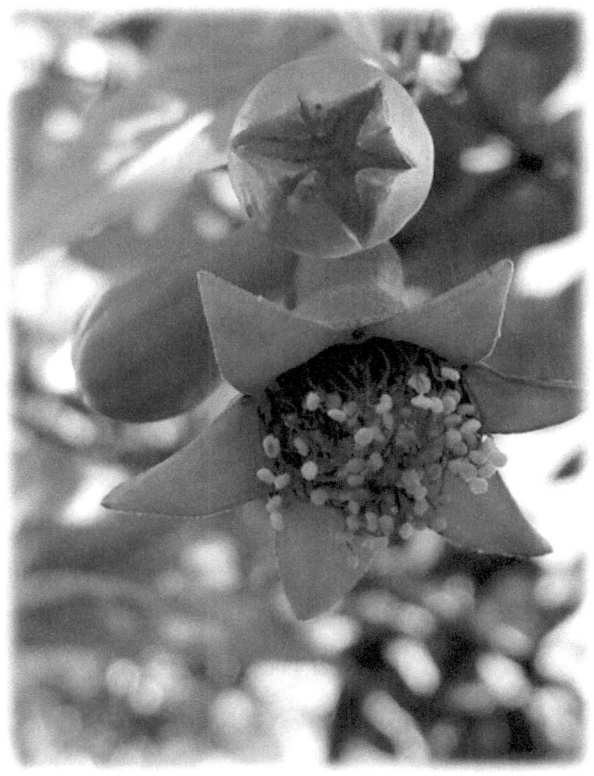

A LITTLE POMEGRANATE SCIENCE FOR YOU

Known by the Latin name *punica granatum ("seeded apple"),* pomegranate fruit can grow on a small, multi-stemmed shrub or even on pomegranate trees that can grow to be almost 30 feet high. The branches of the tree sprout upward then droop down, similar to the water flow of a fountain. Its leaves are narrow, silky and rectangular. They grow and die-off annually.

The tree or bush itself is accented by bright red flowers, so attractive to the eye that many owners of pomegranate plants opt for the fruitless variety just to have access to the pretty flowers. Flowers also grow in orange, white and pink. Pomegranate flowers average a little over an inch in diameter with four or five petals per flower head.

Pomegranate plants are highly adaptable. While they tend to flourish in subtropical conditions where temperatures alternate between warm – cool and dry - wet, pomegranate plants are also drought-proof. Cultivation of the pomegranate tree has spread from the Mediterranean region throughout the Middle East. The plants are also cultivated in:

- Northern India (hence the moniker "Indian apple")
- Central and Southeast Asia
- North Africa and Tropical Africa
- The Bahamas and West Indies
- The Americas

The plant was introduced to Latin America and North America in the middle of the 18th century by Spanish settlers. Today, it is successfully cultivated in the states of Florida, California and Arizona. While fruitless plants can be grown as far north as Washington D.C, the plant fares much better in temperatures over 40 degrees Fahrenheit. Pomegranates can tolerate temperatures as low as 10 degrees Fahrenheit, but in wetter climates, they are prone to fungal infection and rotting.

The fruit of the pomegranate tree ripens six to seven months after the plant flowers. Here in the Northern Hemisphere, pomegranates are generally in season from October to January. In the Southern Hemisphere, the fruit is in season from March through the month of May.

There are several types of pomegranate plants commonly cultivated. The variety planted determines the appearance of the fruit.

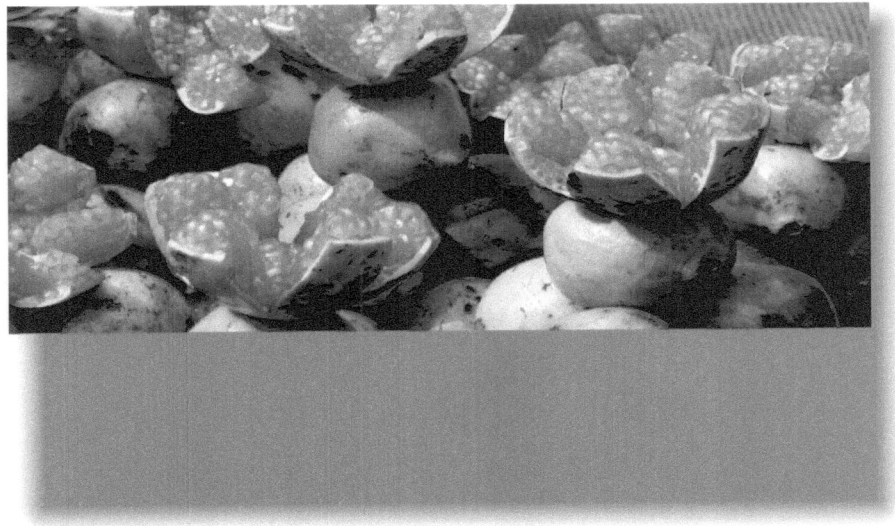

- The **Balegal** tree produces large, pink-skinned pomegranates with fruit that is dark red and very sweet.
- **Crab** varieties produce large, flavorful fruit that have a slightly nutty taste.
- **Cloud** pomegranates are mid-sized fruit with a slightly greenish hue to the skin.

- Cultivated in the West Indies, the **Francis** variety of pomegranate fruit are large and sweet with a tough, thick outer skin.
- **Freshman** pomegranates are large and round, averaging about 3 inches in diameter. The fruit is sweet. Both the skin and the seeds of freshman pomegranates are pink.

HISTORY OF THE FRUIT

Evidence of the pomegranate tree dates back thousands of years. The legend surrounding pomegranate fruit has made its way into all the major religions and popular folklore.

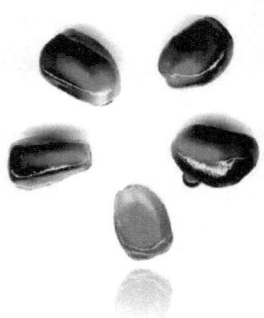

In Greek mythology, after Hades was forced to release the goddess Persephone as his prisoner, he gave her pomegranate seeds. When she later ate the seeds, which she loved, Persephone unknowingly tied herself to the underworld and ended up having to spend one-third of each year in the underworld with Hades. To this day, the pomegranate is commonly used to signify Persephone.

The pomegranate fruit was also used to evoke the presence the Aegean Triple Goddess.

In Judeo-Christian tradition, the use of pomegranates is documented in the Pentateuch in the Book of Exodus as part of the ornamentation for the robe worn by the Hebrew High Priest. Even the design of King Solomon's coronet is said to have been patterned after the pomegranate's calyx.

The Qur'an names pomegranates specifically in the list of good things created by Allah. As well, Islamic scripture reports that pomegranates grow in the gardens of paradise.

In Hinduism, pomegranates are a symbol of fertility and prosperity and associated with at least two deities, namely Bhoomidevi, the earth goddess, and Lord Ganesha, the god of beginnings and success.

Certain North African and Middle Eastern traditions included burial with pomegranates in hopes of being reborn. Ancient Babylonians believed the pomegranate had the power to resurrect life. Famed Egyptian pharaoh Tutankhamun (most commonly known as King Tut) is said to have been buried with pomegranates

Pomegranates made their way into China during the Tang Dynasty, which lasted from 618-907 BCE. At the time, pomegranates – a seeded fruit - were a symbol of fertility and posterity. Drawing of pomegranates were placed in homes as a way of promoting fertility.

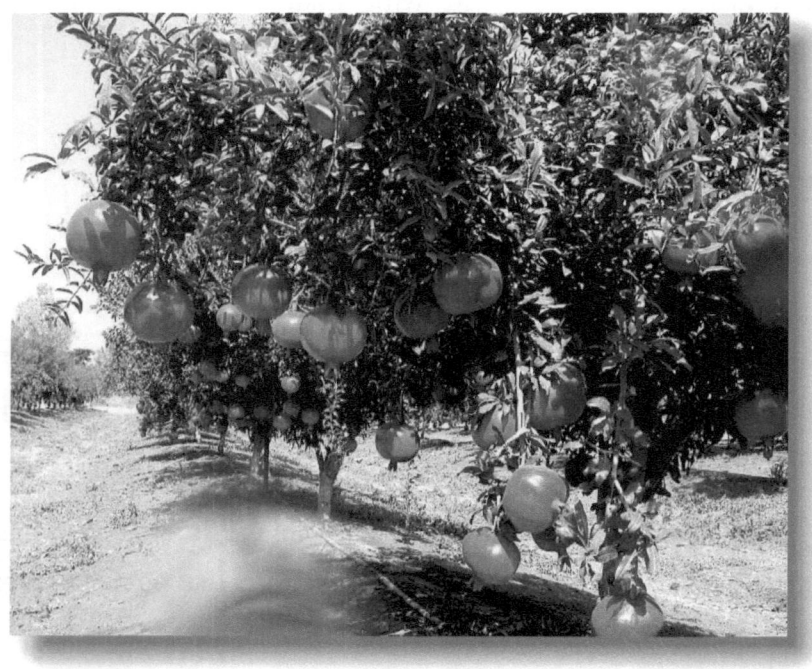

THE POMEGRANATE BUSINESS TODAY

Today, the fruit so deeply entrenched in the rituals and belief systems of religions around the world is yet growing in popularity. In the last ten years, the fruit that is widely believed to promote rebirth has had a rebirth of its own, so to speak. This rebirth is not simply due to an increase in visibility at the grocery store, but also a shift in the way the fruit is marketed.

According to Tom Tjerandsen, manager of the California-based Pomegranate Council, up to half the domestic harvest of pomegranates are expected to be exported to places such as Australia, New Zealand, Canada, Mexico, the European Union and South America.

Those who want to get access to the magical health benefits of pomegranates can do so by getting the fruit, pomegranate supplements and commercially-produced pomegranate juice and spices. In the U.S., pomegranate fruit and pomegranate shrubs are also cultivated for visual appeal because there is a steady demand in the market to use the fruit and plant in seasonal home décor.

In 2002, Pom Wonderful brought the experience of drinking pomegranate juice to the American market at a time when few Westerners had ever tasted the fruit. In anticipation of bringing the product to market, the company allocated tens of millions of dollars to clinical testing in an effort to research and validate the health benefits of pomegranate juice. As well, the company purchased a one hundred and eight-acre pomegranate orchard in California's San Joaquin Valley for domestic cultivation of the fruit. A little over a decade later, Pom Wonderful's pomegranate juice, pomegranate supplement and pre-packaged aril sales trumped $165 million, even amid disputes of deceptive advertising claims brought on by the Federal Trade Commission.

Other pomegranate juice marketers such as Puregranate, PureFresh Sales Inc., Ruby Fresh Pomegranates, Minute Maid and Old Orchard have also seen growth in their pomegranate programs in recent years. Like Pom Wonderful, these companies tout the health benefits of pomegranates and substantiate their marketing claims using both scientific research and the fruit's near-legendary ancient reputation.

PART TWO:

THE POMEGRANATE & YOUR HEALTH

USING POMEGRANATES FOR YOUR HEALTH

Now that we have gotten the background information out of the way, let's get to the good stuff - the actual eating and healing part of the plan.

PICKING A POMEGRANATE

For those who buy pomegranates from the local farmers market or the produce section of the neighborhood grocery store, you can rest in the knowledge that the pomegranates on display are already ripe. No sniffing or squeezing necessary. The chances are pretty good that whatever piece you pick is ready to be eaten. However, you do want to make sure you pick the best-looking fruit.

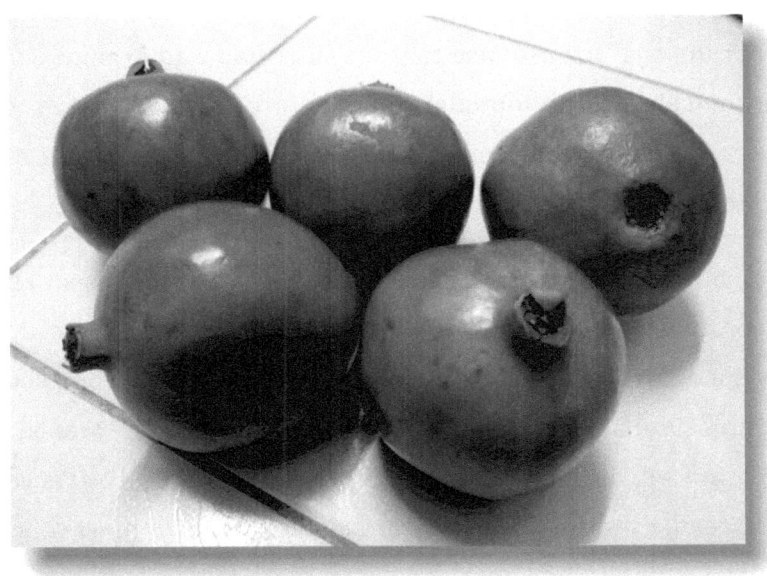

Pick a pomegranate that is uniformly colored all over with minimal brown spots (a sign of over-exposure to the sun). Pomegranates can range in color from pink to burgundy, depending on the variety of the fruit itself. The skin of your pomegranate should be tight. Typically, the skin of a pomegranate is leathery, but look for fruit with a smooth leather look, not bunched or wrinkled. If the skin looks a little wrinkled, it's probably dehydrated and the fruit will not be as juicy.

Also, avoid pomegranates that are bruised, cut or showing signs of rot. Don't get me wrong. The skin is thick enough and strong enough to withstand a little wear and tear. The pomegranate is especially well-suited for storage. Its thick skin provides a built-in cushion for safe packaging. Once ripened, pomegranates are clipped close to the base of the fruit to prevent unnecessary damage from the stem during transport.

It's not unusual for produce to get a little knocked around or spend time outside of its optimal temperature storage range during transport. So go ahead and inspect your fruit to make sure it looks good to you.

Once you get your pomegranates home, you can store them at room temperature for about a week before they will either need to be consumed or refrigerated. Pomegranates have a rather long shelf life. The pomegranate maintains both its flavor and appearance when stored in cool, dark places at temperatures of 32º to 41º Fahrenheit. At this temperature, stored pomegranate can keep for more than half a year and maintain its flavor as long as the air stays between 80% to

85% humidity. Just a 5% increase in humidity would cut the shelf life of a pomegranate by more than half.

REMOVING THE ARILS FROM A POMEGRANATE

One look at an opened pomegranate and you can probably foresee a mess in your future. That's because the arils (the average pomegranate has between 600 and 1,000 of them) are filled with red pulp and if enough pressure is applied, one or more of the hundreds of arils in your pomegranate will pop, spilling that delicious red juice.

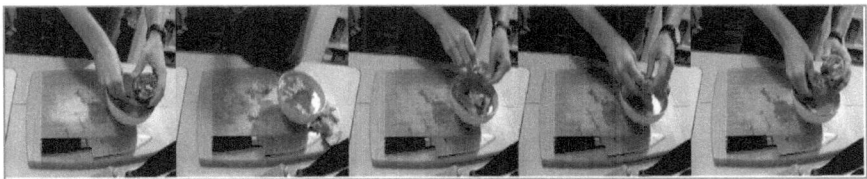

There is definitely an art to eating a pomegranate. Improper technique can leave cleaning up a sticky mess or worse, trying to rid your clothes, furniture and any nearby fabrics of stains. I've listed a few no-mess methods for removing and enjoying the arils of a pomegranate. Trust me. It's worth the effort.

SPATULA METHOD

1. Use a sharp knife to cut your pomegranate in half.
2. Fill a medium-sized bowl to the halfway point with cold water.

3. Hold your pomegranate over the bowl of cold water and turn the fruit cut side down.

4. Use a wooden spatula to firmly tap the rounded bottom of the pomegranate to loosen the arils. This method takes a little longer than the previous method but delivers the same result.

Here are two cool videos I found that show how to cut and get the seeds out of Pomegranate the easiest way.

https://www.youtube.com/watch?v=HGYpk395PUA

https://www.youtube.com/watch?v=aUsfw-KppCU

UNDERWATER METHOD

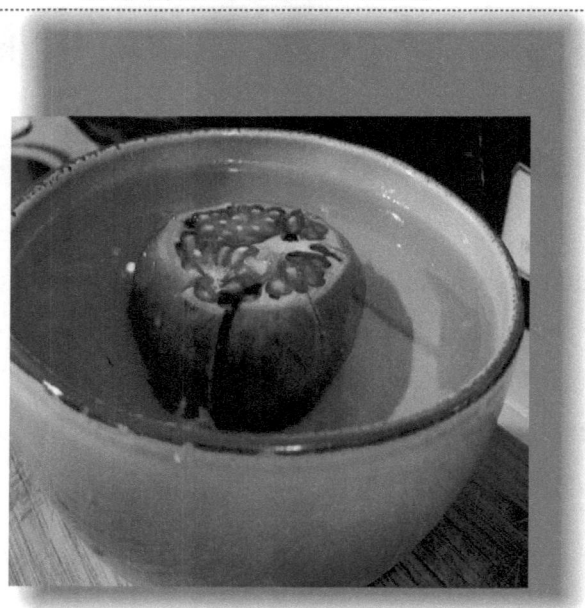

1. Use a sharp knife to cut your pomegranate into quarters.

2. Fill a large bowl to the halfway point with cold water and submerge the entire pomegranate in the water.

3. Bend back the rind of a single wedge to expose the arils.

4. While keeping the fruit underwater, gently use your fingers to separate the arils from the membranes. Detached membranes are lightweight and will float to the top of the bowl. Your pomegranate arils are heavier and will settle at the bottom of the bowl.

5. Slowly pour the water out of the bowl being careful not to spill your newly-separated pomegranate arils.

6. If necessary, gently dry the arils using several pieces of absorbent paper towel.

Once you have successful separated your arils, you can eat them as you would any other snack or add them to other foods. Arils will keep for up to three days if bagged and refrigerated.

HOW TO JUICE A POMEGRANATE

In recent years, the popularity of raw and bottled pomegranate juice has grown in the West. In fact, there's a pretty good chance you'll find some yourself the next time you visit the juice section of the produce department. Pomegranate juice is a fantastic source of vitamin C and antioxidants. When shopping for bottled juice, however, make sure to buy 100% pomegranate juice with no added sugars.

If you prefer fresh juice, you can take advantage of a few handy techniques to help you easily extract juice from your pomegranates.

BLENDER METHOD

1. Use either the underwater method or the spatula method to separate the arils from the membranes. Do not include membranes in your juice. It makes the juice bitter and extremely dry-tasting (from the astringent properties of the membranes).

2. Add 2 cups of arils to the bottom of a blender. Pulse the arils a few times just to break up the seeds and separate some of the juice.

3. Sit a mesh strainer over your glass or container and pour the mixture through the strainer. Let the juice drain from the strainer.

4. Use the rounded bottom of a tablespoon to firmly press more juice from the seeds through the strainer and into your container.

Here is a very popular video I found on the blender method, take a look

https://www.youtube.com/watch?v=VzvsQVIX0mY

JUICER METHOD

1. Cut a medium-sized pomegranate in half. Remove the membrane.

2. If using a hand-press juicer, press the juice from the arils into a separate container by pressing and twisting the juicer into the pomegranate half. If using an electric juicer, use the spatula method or the underwater method to separate arils from the rind and membrane. Then pour 2 cups of arils into the juicer and run the juicer until no more juice runs out.

3. Pass the juice through a cheesecloth or mesh strainer to remove seeds.

Here is a infomercial video of a juicer that shows how to use a juicer to juice Pomegranate. This is how I juice it.

https://www.youtube.com/watch?v=NzbVlJr78TA

ROLLING METHOD

1. Wash a medium-sized pomegranate and put it in a plastic freezer bag.

2. Use the palm of your hand to firmly roll the pomegranate against a hard surface like a table or countertop.

3. You will hear the arils pop on the inside of the fruit. Keep rolling the fruit until you stop hearing the arils pop.

4. Once you are satisfied you have broken all the arils, slice the top off your fruit and pour the juice in a container.

Fresh pomegranate juice can keep for up to three days if refrigerated and up to six months if frozen.

Here is a video on how to use the rolling method

https://www.youtube.com/watch?v=rLrAhvlqfKY

THE HEALING EFFECTS OF POMEGRANATE

By far, one of the most impressive things about the pomegranate has to be its nutrient-density. Pomegranates provide the uncommon benefit of being both delicious and highly nutritious. That means you won't have to dress up the fruit in order to get kids to eat it. In that regard, it's tasty enough to stand on its own.

THE POMEGRANATE AS SUPER FOOD

So, what qualifies the pomegranate as a super food? Well, pomegranates are high in fiber, vitamin C, B-complex vitamins and antioxidants. They also have notable amounts of vitamin A, vitamin E, vitamin K, manganese, potassium, copper, calcium, beta carotene, iron and protein. Here are just a few quick nutritional facts you may not have known about the pomegranate:

10 NUTRITIONAL FACTS OF POMEGRANATE

1. The pomegranate has more antioxidants than red wine, grape juice and green tea and does a better job of protecting your cells from free radicals.

2. One medium-sized pomegranate delivers about 40% of the recommended daily dose of vitamin C.

3. A pomegranate with a diameter of just three inches can pack 25% of your daily folate requirement. Folate is a water-soluble B vitamin (B9) that promotes the

production of red blood cells and supports nerve function. Folate also helps prevent anemia and dementia.

4. A pomegranate of that size will also contain about 10% of your B6 (pyridoxine) for the day. Vitamin B6 helps the body to metabolize amino acids, glucose and lipids in the liver.

5. A pomegranate four inches in diameter offers around 5 grams of protein and 11 grams of soluble and insoluble dietary fiber – that's 45% of your recommended daily fiber.

6. The pomegranate also provides about 5% of your daily potassium.

7. Pomegranates have antioxidant properties. Antioxidants help inhibit the oxidation and deterioration of your body's cells and prevents the attack of damaged, oxidized cells (free radicals) on your body's healthy cells.

8. Pomegranates have antiviral properties. They help slow, inhibit and destroy viruses that could lead to disease.

9. Pomegranates have antibacterial / antibiotic properties. They help slow and kill the growth of harmful bacteria.

10. Pomegranate seeds are also anti-inflammatory to reduce swelling.

A good way to understand the nutritional value of the pomegranate is to take a look at the value of the fruit's individual offerings.

14 ESSENTIAL VITAMINS AND MINERALS OF POMEGRANATE ARILS

The edible pulp know as arils contain the majority of the pomegranate's nutritional value. The arils include both the tiny seeds and the juice sac surrounding each seed. The arils are responsible for the fruit's high fiber content as well as its supply of vitamins and minerals. Pomegranate arils are known to have strong disease fighting properties.

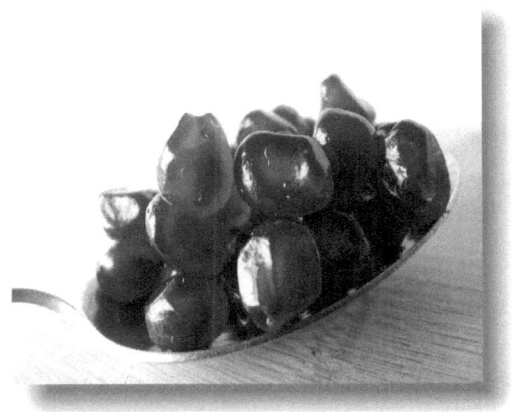

1. Beta Carotene – Beta carotene is a powerful antioxidant that converts to vitamin A in the intestines.

2. Calcium – Calcium is a vital mineral needed by your body for bone and muscle health. Calcium deficiencies

can contribute to stunted growth in children and low bone density in adults.

3. Copper – It probably doesn't get anywhere near the press it should, but copper impacts your health in a variety of ways. Sufficient amounts of copper are needed for your bone health, maintaining a proper balance of red and white blood cells, healthy eyes, reducing cholesterol and controlling skin pigmentation. Copper also has anti-inflammatory properties.

4. Fiber – Heart-healthy fiber supports your digestive system by moving food through the body more quickly. Fiber also helps to lower bad cholesterol and regulate blood sugar levels.

5. Iron – Iron helps in the production of hemoglobin, which carries oxygen through your blood and throughout your entire body. Say goodbye to anemia.

6. Manganese – This mineral helps the body to absorb several B vitamins. It also has antioxidant properties, promotes nerve and thyroid health, helps regulate blood sugar levels and reduces bad cholesterol.

7. Potassium – Potassium helps your muscles contract and your body to maintain normal blood pressure. This is especially important for your heart health.

8. Protein – Protein molecules are needed to maintain, build and replace the body's tissues. This includes muscles, the body's systems and organs.

9. Vitamin A – Vitamin A is an immune system booster. It has antibacterial and antiviral properties, slows down tumor growth and promotes the growth of healthy cells.

10. Vitamin B5 – Also known as pantothenic acid, this vitamin helps your body metabolize energy and maintain proper sodium and potassium levels. B5 is essential in helping your body to regulate its fluids. That includes both cell moisture and blood pressure.

11. Vitamin B6 – Vitamin B6 is one of those vitamins we don't seem to get enough of in the typical American diet but B6 is important. It aids in metabolism, tissue repair, cell production and the production of antibodies needed to fight disease.

12. Vitamin C – There's no shortage of foods rich and vitamin C, nor foodstuffs fortified with vitamin C and for good reason. Vitamin C is an immune system booster. It's essential in protecting the body from a host of diseases and dysfunctions from the common cold to heart disease.

13. Vitamin E – This antioxidant protects the body from environmental toxins and cellular deconstruction. It

helps skin to heal faster and is often added to cosmetics for its rejuvenating properties.

14. Vitamin K – Vitamin K is important for bone and heart health. It helps your bones to absorb and hang on to calcium. Vitamin K is instrumental in helping the blood to clot.

ESSENTIAL AND HEALTHY POMEGRANATE SEED OIL

Pomegranate seed oil is made from the distilled essential oil of the pomegranate seed. The oil is lightweight, amber-colored and has a soft, fruity scent.

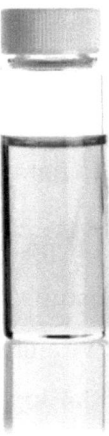

Pure pomegranate oil is rather expensive. You can probably imagine it takes quite a few pomegranates (200 pounds or so) to create even one pound of oil. You can expect to pay at least $10 for an ounce of this oil, but that ounce will go a long way. Unlike most essential oils, pomegranate oil can be administered topically or orally and is a popular additive in cosmetics, drinks and nutritional supplements.

HEALING POWER OF POMEGRANATE SEED OIL

Part of what makes this oil so valuable is it provides a hefty supply of benefits to your body's largest protective organ – the skin. Pomegranate seed oil is a fantastic resource for overall skin care as well as a strengthener for hair and nails. It is a moisturizer that helps skin to retain its youthful glow and elasticity, which minimizes the appearance of fine lines and wrinkles. Pomegranate seed oil promotes skin cell regeneration. It is also high in antioxidants so it protects the skin cells from being destroyed by free radical damage.

The anti-inflammatory and antimicrobial properties of pomegranate oil help the skin to maintain the proper pH balance and fight off infections and skin damage, which promotes proper skin healing and minimizes the effects of eczema, dry skin, skin rashes, and sun burn. It also decreases the frequency and severity of acne lesions. Pomegranate oil also has astringent qualities which help to tighten and firm the skin.

Pomegranate oil is also high in phytoestrogens. Phytoestrogens are naturally-occurring, plant-derived female hormones that are not produced internally, but are consumed. Phytoestrogens have been associated with lowered risk of menopausal symptoms (including hot flashes, mood swings, loss of appetite, and night sweats), heart disease, breast cancer and osteoporosis.

Pomegranate extract is often a combination of the pomegranate juice, seeds, peel, stem and flower. The extract can be purchased in pill, capsule or powder form and provides a wide range of health benefits that combine the collective powers of pomegranate arils and the seed oil along with the healing powers of pomegranate peel.

Despite the fact that the bulk of research regarding the health benefits of the pomegranate has been focused on the pulp of the fruit, the pomegranate peel has been used in traditional medicine for centuries. In fact, scientists from the Institute of Hygiene and Environmental Medicine in Tianjin, China report the peel of the pomegranate has double the amount of antioxidants as the fruit.

The astringent properties of the pomegranate peel can also be used to stop bleeding in many parts of the body. This includes nose bleeds, bleeding gums and excessive menstrual bleeding. Rind powder helps to reduce inflammation associated with arthritis and is a great source of beta carotene, potassium, calcium and phosphorus.

*** Be careful. Pomegranate rind has health benefits, but it also contains toxins that may be dangerous for the delicate systems of small children and pregnant women. Drinking the juice and eating the fruit is fine, but small children and pregnant women should not take pomegranate extract or supplements. ***

Researchers have found the antioxidants in pomegranate flowers are two to three times more potent than those found in green tea and red wine. Imagine that! Extract from these flowers is believed to aid in food digestion, remedy diarrhea and promote weight loss by suppressing the appetite. Pomegranate flower extract is also shown to help maintain heart health in patients with type 2 diabetes.

Throughout the ages, the uses for pomegranates have included everything from birth control to fighting cancer. Between traditional medicine and today's modern research-based science, you can create a virtual catalog of ailments and coinciding pomegranate remedies.

Now, there are government agencies in place whose job it is to protect the interest of the general public by deciding how food and drug products can be marketed and distributed. The Food and Drug Administration has strict requirements on what manufacturers and marketers can claim a product does and what they cannot claim. As such, you will often find that supplement marketers tend to steer clear of making any medical claims that can be perceived as deceptive by the Food and Drug Administration even if those claims are true.

So this next section is organized in way that provides you with a list of ailments and ways pomegranates **_may_** serve to either relieve or treat those ailments. Again, this book is not a medical manual. In fact, if you are suffering from any ailment at all, I would advise you to seek the guidance of a reputable medical provider in your community. Also be aware that pomegranate juice, while mostly harmless, can interfere with the effectiveness of some prescribed drug treatments. So be sure to talk to your doctor before adding pomegranate juice or extracts to your daily nutrition plan.

The American Cancer Society estimated there would be more than 1.6 million new cancer cases diagnosed in 2013 and more than 580,000 cancer-related deaths just in the U.S. alone. That means nearly one-quarter of all deaths that take place in the country will be caused by cancer. That's a sobering reality. Now the interesting thing to note is research demonstrates 80% – 90% of all cancers are related to environmental factors and 30% – 40% are directly linked to diet. It makes sense that if your diet can cause you to get cancer, your diet can also prevent cancer.

Pomegranates are believed to help in the fight against cancer. The American Association for Cancer Research reports drinking at least 2 ounces of pomegranate juice a day can improve prostate health. Researchers at the University of Maryland Medical Center believe the antioxidants in pomegranates have the ability to disrupt the cycle of cancerous cell growth in men battling prostate cancer.

The antioxidants present in pomegranate juice can help reduce the risk of developing cancer in the first place and may also help fight existing cancer cells (including prostate cancer, breast cancer, lymphoma and benign prostatic hyperplasia) in the body. In men with prostate cancer, drinking 8 ounces of pomegranate seed extract daily is known to quadruple the time it takes cancer cells to double, thus decreasing the risk of the patient dying from the disease. One study on record noted the doubling time for cancerous cells in men who drank pomegranate extract went from 15 months to 54 months.

Pomegranate extract can also reduce the size of a tumor by slowing the supply of blood sent to it. The antioxidant properties of pomegranate extract are believed to decrease one's chances of developing skin cancer by actively fighting against the formation of cancerous lesions.

HIGH CHOLESTEROL

I can't say enough about the role antioxidants play in your health. Specifically when we talk about pomegranates, antioxidants are a BIG DEAL. Antioxidants are concentrated so much more in pomegranate juice than in other fruit juices. This is good news for your arteries.

If you're wondering if pomegranate juice can lower your cholesterol, the answer is yes and no. Antioxidants help to slow the build-up of cholesterol in your arteries. So pomegranate juice works by slowing the accumulation of low-density lipoprotein, also known as LDL (bad cholesterol). It's not necessarily that the cholesterol currently in your body is going to decrease with every glass you drink. It's that pomegranate juice will slow down the plaque-building process. Researchers at Technion Institute in Israel published a report which proved patients with clogged arteries who drank pomegranate juice had less arterial plaque growth.

DIGESTIVE SYSTEM DISORDER

Pomegranate has been used for years to treat digestive problems. Pomegranate tea is used to treat a variety of stomach ailments including diarrhea, dysentery, cholera and upset stomach. The rind of a pomegranate is used to help expel parasites from the intestines.

GUM DISEASE

The astringent, antiviral and antibacterial properties of pomegranate peel have been used for years to deal with the symptoms of gum disease. Pomegranate rind powder is even used in the preparation of some toothpastes and tooth powders. In recent years, Thai researchers have found pomegranate helps fight the buildup of the microorganisms responsible for plaque that can lead to gum disease.

The researchers also found that pomegranate in conjunction with the herb gotu kola were able to decrease the gap and restore the attachment between the gums and teeth just by inserting chips containing the extracts between the tooth and gum line. The powder from pomegranate peel can also be used to remedy bad breath when taken with water twice a day.

HARDENING OF THE ARTERIES

There is evidence to suggest drinking pomegranate juice helps to improve blood flow to the heart. We talked a bit about pomegranate's blood-building properties. The iron content helps the blood deliver oxygen all over the body. The antioxidants slow down the buildup of LDL cholesterol. Pomegranate's antioxidant and anti-inflammatory properties also keep your arteries from being thick and stiff and reverses carotid atherosclerosis (the hardening of the arteries) by reducing oxidative stress and inflammation in the blood vessels.

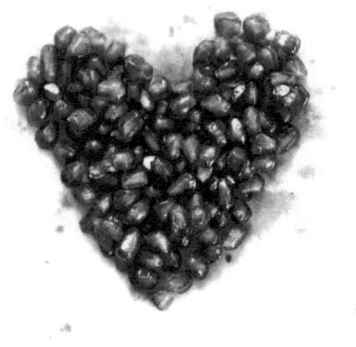

The American Heart Association defines heart disease as the series of heart-related ailments that result from atherosclerosis (plaque buildup that narrows the arteries, slows the flow of blood and hardens the walls of the arteries making them inflexible). This includes heart attacks, stroke, heart failure, arrhythmias and heart valve problems.

Daily doses of pomegranate juice will do several things to promote a healthy heart. First, pomegranate juice reduces the rate at which plaque builds up in the arteries. Next, it helps to make your blood flow a seamless process. Third, pomegranate juice sends much-needed oxygen to the heart to help ensure it continues pumping. Next, it loads your body with potassium to promote muscle contraction and help maintain normal blood pressure. Together, this cocktail of heart-healthy actions helps to reduce your risk of heart attack and heart disease altogether.

When you launch into a weight loss plan in the ongoing fight against obesity, think of the pomegranate as a fantastic substitute for any and every fat-laced alternative. While a juice fast is never recommended as a way to lose weight, abstaining from certain foods in order to bring your body back in balance is always a good idea and should be done at least twice a year.

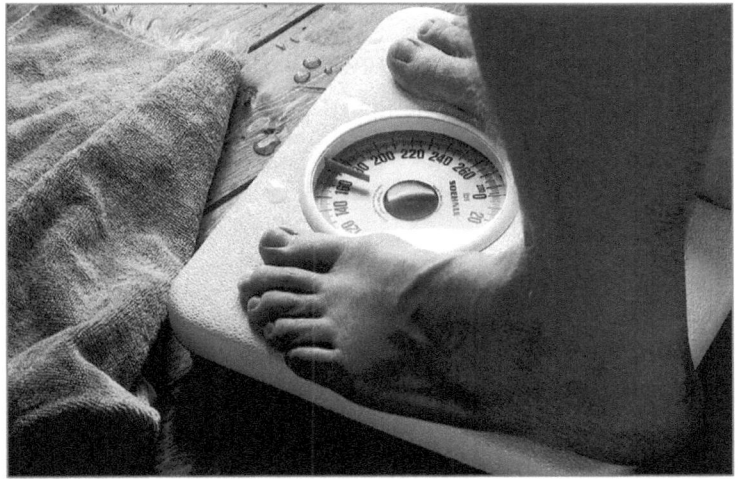

Because the pomegranate is so nutrient-rich and trumps other fruit in antioxidant content, it's the ideal low-calorie replacement option for any refined sugars or high-fat foods you may be removing from your diet whether temporarily or long term. In the spring and summer months, you may have to opt for a serving of bottled juice when the fruit is not in season. Don't fret. There is plenty of bottled pomegranate juice to go around. Just make sure you are getting 100% pure pomegranate juice with no added sugars.

A study conducted by researchers in the Department of Biological Sciences and Biotechnology at Tsinghua University in Beijing showed a decrease in the absorption of fat in laboratory mice who were administered pomegranate leaf extract. The extract also worked as an effective appetite suppressant.

OTHER AILMENTS

To get a better grasp on the vastness of the benefits provided by pomegranates, take a look at this list of uses. Most of these remedies have been used for centuries with practitioners of traditional medicine.

ALZHEIMER'S DISEASE – Pomegranate seed extract is believed to support neurological functions and reduce the risk of Alzheimer's disease in elderly people.

BREASTS – Sagging ones, that is. The astringents present in pomegranate oil are the perfect remedy to help perk up sagging breasts.

CATARACTS – Certain varieties of pomegranate juice are used as eyedrops to slow or prevent cataracts.

COMMON COLD – Peel the membranes from pomegranate arils and set those membranes aside for later use to get relief from the symptoms of the common cold. Steep them in tea or eat them plain.

CONTRACEPTION – In Ancient Greece, pomegranates were used as a form of contraception. Research today provides evidence to support the ancient practice of using a pomegranate pessary (vaginal suppository) for birth control. In fact, modern studies show this method of birth control reduced fertility in female rats by 50% and in female guinea pigs by 100%. Fertility was restored some forty days after the pessary stopped being used.

COUGH SUPPRESSANT – Sucking on a pomegranate peel or taking small amounts of pomegranate paste (made from the peel and water) can help relieve your cough and clear your chest.

ERECTILE DYSFUNCTION – Research conducted by the Journal of Impotence Research corroborated the long-held belief that pomegranate juice can help improve erections. Pure pomegranate juice is said to increase sperm count and semen quality.

HEMORRHOIDS – Pomegranate peel steeped in hot water can be used as a topical remedy for hemorrhoid flare-ups.

HERPES – The immunity boosting power of pomegranates coupled with its high concentration of antioxidants makes it a good tool for blocking herpes despite the fact that pomegranates are an acidic food. Pomegranate extract can help to minimize the ability of the virus to replicate, which shortens the duration of outbreaks.

IMMUNE SYSTEM – Pomegranate seed oil is believed to fortify the immune system, enabling us to be better equipped to fight diseases like cancer, obesity, diabetes and heart disease.

MENOPAUSE – Pomegranate oil helps minimize the physical and emotional symptoms of menopause. Women have been known to take pomegranate extract to combat depression that may result from the onset of menopause and to reduce the effects of fatigue.

OSTEOARTHRITIS – Researchers believe antioxidants called flavonols help minimize the inflammation that wears down joint cartilage, thereby relieving and even eliminating osteoarthritis.

PREGNANCY – For years, pregnant women have consumed pomegranate juice as a way to prevent premature childbirth and remedy the problem of low birth weight babies. As recently as 2005, Pediatric Research published a study which indicates pomegranate juice may help reduce brain injuries in babies born prematurely.

SORE THROAT – Pomegranate extract added to warm water is used as a gargle for sore throats.

SIDE EFFECTS AND SAFETY PRECAUTIONS

We talked a bit before about the need to exercise some caution in using the pomegranate for nutrition. There are some precautions I want you to be aware of when choosing whether to eat pomegranates, drink the juice, take supplements or use extracts.

INTERACTIONS WITH MEDICATIONS

If you are taking certain types of medications, you may already have received a warning from your physician about juices that may interact with prescribed treatments. In addition to grapefruit juice, black mulberry, wild grape and black raspberry, pomegranate juice can make certain medications less potent than they would be if taken with water.

Avoid pomegranate juice, supplements and extracts if you are taking any of the following medications:

AVOID POMEGRANATE IF YOU TAKE THESE 4 TYPES OF MEDICINES

- ACE Inhibitors are used to control high blood pressure, treat heart disease and prevent kidney damage in diabetes patients. Avoid mixing pomegranate products with Benazepril (Lotensin), Captopril (Capoten), Enalapril (Vasotec), Fosinopril (Monopril), Lisinopril (Zestril) or Ramipril (Altace).

- Blood pressure medications are designed to regulate blood pressure. Well, that is also a function pomegranates perform naturally. Taking pomegranate in addition to taking medications to lower blood pressure may result in low blood pressure.

- Statins are used to lower cholesterols. If you are taking statins, avoid pomegranate products as they may interact with Atorvastatin (Lipitor), Fluvastatin (Lescol), Lovastatin (Mevacor), Pravastatin (Pravachol), Rosuvastatin (Crestor) or Simvastatin (Zocor).

- Warfarin (Coumadin) is a blood thinner. Taking this medication with pomegranate products may cause the blood thinning abilities of warfarin to increase your risk of bleeding.

Exercise caution in consuming and using pomegranate skin. While pomegranate skin contains high amounts of antioxidants, it also contains tannic acid, which is slightly toxic and can be dangerous if ingested excessively. Overall, however, the toxicity levels of the pomegranate are relatively low. Of course, as previously discussed, pregnant women are well-advised to steer clear of anything that contains pomegranate rind or pomegranate stem.

The fastest way to jumpstart a new nutritional plan is to get the information you need along with a few tools to get you started. This time, those tools will come in the form of recipes. I've included ten tasty, low-calorie recipes (plus a little something extra for Mom and Dad) to help you incorporate pomegranates successfully into your everyday life.

Sure, it's great to sit down with a handful of seeds and just snack between meals, but a little creativity can go a long way toward helping you to really cement the habit of including pomegranates as part of your daily diet. The recipes are simple, tasty with a touch of international flare here and there. No worries. You'll love them.

*   *   *   *

POMEGRANATE MOLASSES

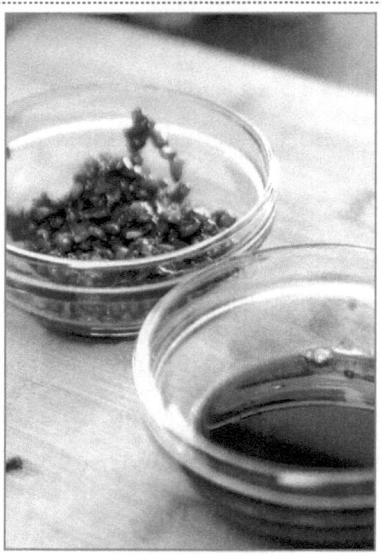

6 cups of 100% pure pomegranate juice
1 cup of brown sugar
4 teaspoons of lemon juice
1 16-oz Mason jar

1. Combine all ingredients in a large saucepan and cook over medium heat, stirring with a large wooden spoon.
2. Once the sugar has completely dissolved, reduce your heat to low and cook for 60 to 90 minutes. Your molasses will cook down

from 6 cups of juice to about 2 cups of thick syrup.

3. Once the molasses is done, allow it to cook for about 30 minutes then pour the contents into your mason jar for future use.

RUBY SALSA

Arils from 2 medium pomegranates (about 1 cup of arils)
1/8 cup of finely chopped sweet onions
1/4 cup of chopped red bell peppers
1/8 cup of diced peaches
1/4 cup of steak tomatoes chunks
1 tablespoon of lime juice

1. Remove the arils from the pomegranate and place them in a mesh strainer over a container.
2. Use the rounded bottom of a spoon to gently mash the arils to release some of the juice into the container.
3. Pour your ingredients including the pomegranate juice into a mixing bowl and mix the ingredients together by hand.
4. Cover and chill for at least 30 minutes before using.
5.

POMEGRANATE FIZZ

1 cup of low fat plain Greek yogurt (about 6 ounces)
The arils from 1 medium pomegranate (about ½ cup)
½ tablespoon of agave nectar
1 teaspoon of flaxseeds
¼ cup of almond milk
4 ice cubes

1. This is an easy one. Just toss all of your ingredients in a blender and blend for about 30 seconds.

GOAT CHEESE AND POMEGRANATE CREPES

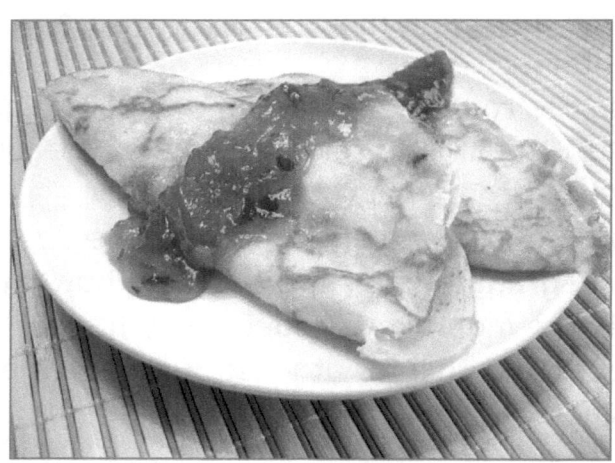

2 cups of all-purpose flour

4 eggs
1 tablespoon of crushed almonds
1 cup of almond milk
1 cup of water
1/2 teaspoon of kosher salt
4 tablespoons of butter, melted
1 cup of pomegranate molasses
1 cup of pomegranate arils
2 cups of goat cheese
1/8 cup of heavy whipping cream

1. In a medium mixing bowl, use a hand mixer to mix the goat cheese and whipping cream. Blend until creamy. Let sit.
2. In a large mixing bowl, use an electric hand mixer to mix the flour, almonds and the eggs. Next add your almond milk, water, salt and butter.
3. Use a griddle or large pan to heat a tablespoon of olive oil. Pour a thin layer of batter onto the hot griddle. Cover the entire bottom of the griddle, but keep the layer thin.
4. Cook the crepe on the first side for 90 seconds. Loosen the edges with a spatula and flip. Cook the other side for another 30 seconds.
5. Plate your crepe. Scoop a generous amount of the goat cheese and whipping cream mixture onto the crepe and sprinkle pomegranate arils on top before loosely

rolling your crepe and fixing with one toothpick on each end.

6. Drizzle pomegranate molasses on the crepe and enjoy hot.

KISIR

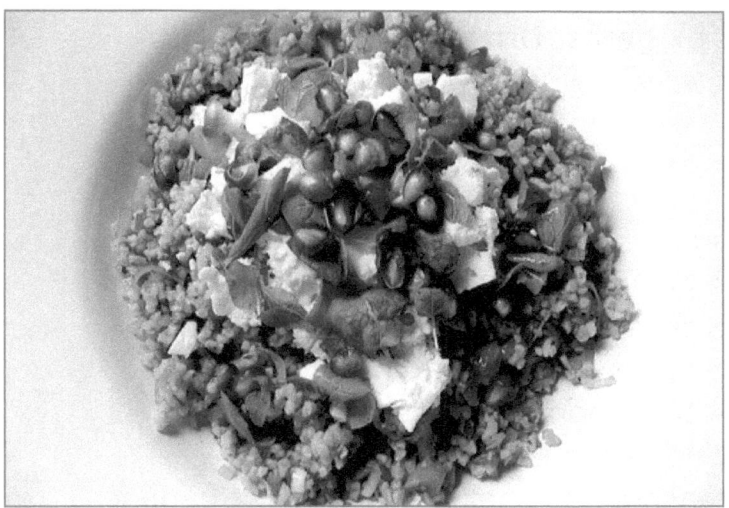

8 ounces of bulgur wheat

2 Vidalia onions, finely chopped

6 ounces of cherry tomatoes chopped

1 ounce of finely chopped toasted walnuts

3 tablespoons of fresh herbs (mint & parsley)

1 tablespoon of olive oil

1 cup of feta cheese

1 cup of pomegranate arils

1. Put your bulgur in a large bowl and pour in boiling water. Let it sit covered for five minutes. Once the time has passed,

uncover the bulgur, fluff with a fork and let it cool.
2. Stir in walnuts, tomatoes and onions. Garnish with feta cheese, pomegranate herbs. Drizzle with olive oil.
3.

BUTTERNUT SQUASH

---

1 small sweet onion diced
1/4 cup finely chopped celery
1/8 teaspoon fresh, chopped thyme
1/8 teaspoon dried thyme
1/4 teaspoon dried rosemary
1 fresh sage leaf, finely chopped
1 teaspoon kosher salt and black pepper
1 tablespoon olive oil
1 small butternut squash, peeled and cubed
1 1/3 cups chicken stock
1/2 cup heavy cream
1/2 cup pomegranate arils
Sour cream

1. Use a large saucepan to cook vegetables and herbs in olive oil over medium heat for 5 to 7 minutes, until onions are translucent. Add salt and pepper. Cook an additional 2 to 3 minutes.
2. Add the squash and chicken stock to the pan. Allow mixture to cook covered on medium low heat for 20 minutes.

3. When squash is tender, pour the mixture in a blender and puree or pulse until the soup is smooth. Return the mixture to the saucepan and add heavy cream.
4. Serve bisque hot, garnished with sour cream and pomegranate arils.

PORK MEDALLIONS WITH POMEGRANATE MOLASSES

1 pork tenderloin, approximately 12 ounces
1 teaspoon of lemon pepper
1 pound of broccoli
1 tablespoon of pomegranate molasses
1 teaspoon of olive oil
1/4 cup of maple or honey mustard
1/2 cup of chicken stock
1/2 cup of chopped walnuts
1 tablespoons lard

1. Heat olive oil in a large skillet. Start at the thickest part of the tenderloin and cut each piece across into 2 inch-wide pieces. Do this for every piece but the last piece where it narrows. Fold the last piece in half and secure it with a toothpick so it is about the same thickness as the others. Season with lemon pepper. Add pork to skillet. Increase heat to medium-high and cook 3 minutes.
2. Pour 2 cups of hot water in a large saucepan. Cover and cook on high heat. Add broccoli to boiling water. Cover and cook 3 to 5 minutes to the firmness of your choice.
3. Turn medallions over and lower heat to medium. Cook the other side of the pork for another 3 to 5 minutes. Mix pomegranate

molasses, mustard and chicken stock in small bowl.

4. Add stock mixture and walnuts to skillet. Cover cook on high heat. Then uncover plate pork. Stir sauce to mix well and let reduce just a little. Pour the sauce over your pork medallions.

5. While sauce thickens, drain broccoli in colander. Put butter in saucepan over

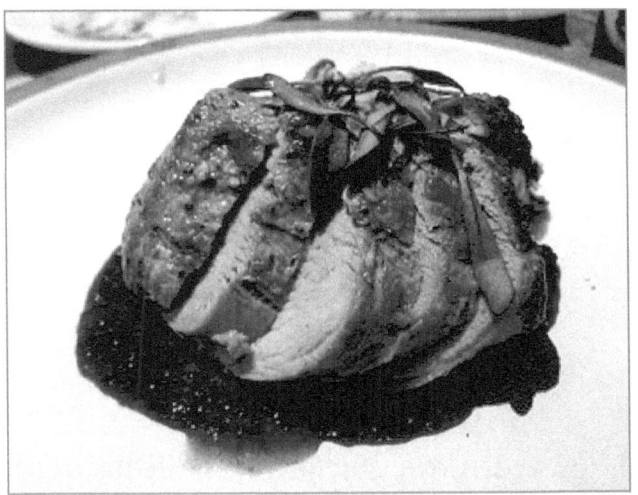

medium-high heat. Add broccoli and stir gently 1 minute. Serve broccoli with pork.

SPICY CHICKEN TACOS WITH RUBY SALSA

1 cup of ruby salsa
2 pounds of boneless skinless chicken thighs
1 cup of chicken broth
1/8 cup of crushed jalapenos
1/4 cup cilantro, chopped
Corn or flour tortillas
1 cup of chopped iceberg lettuce
1 cup of shredded sharp cheddar cheese
1 teaspoon of chili powder

1. Remove excess fat from chicken and cut chicken into small cubes.
2. Bring chicken broth to a boil in a medium sauces pan. Add in crushed jalapenos. Once the mixture is boiling, add the chicken then reduce to medium heat and let the mixture cook 20 minutes.
3. Plate the chicken and let it cool for at least ten minutes.
4. Using the remaining chicken broth, create a second mixture of chicken, broth and chili powder and allow it to simmer for another 10 minutes then let it cool for 5 minutes.

Fill each taco shell with chicken, cheese, lettuce and ruby salsa.

POMPOPZ

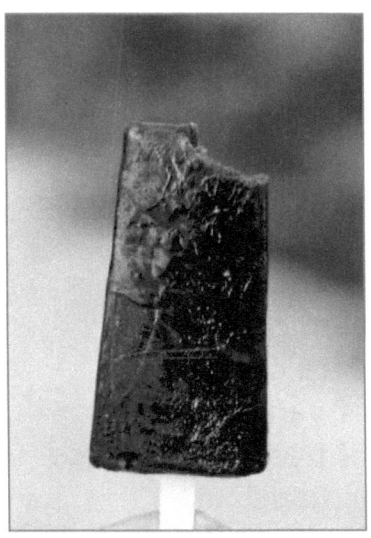

1 cup of fresh sweet blueberries
2 cup of frozen strawberries in syrup
1 cups of almond milk
1 cup of pomegranate juice
1/3 cup pomegranate molasses
1/4 cup water

1. Cook blueberries, strawberries (with syrup), water and molasses on medium high heat in a medium-sized pot.
2. When the mixture begins to boil, stir in almond milk and reduce the heat. Let the mixture cook for 10 to 15 minutes.

3. When the mixture is boiling once again, remove it from the heat and add the cup of pomegranate juice. Use a spatula or fork to mix the liquids together.
4. Allow the mixture to cool for 20 minutes before pouring into ice pop molds to freeze for at least six hours.

POMEGRANATE RICOTTA CHEESECAKE

1 1/2 cups of pomegranate arils
1 pound of cream cheese
1 pound of ricotta cheese
1 tablespoon of vanilla extract
1 tablespoon of fresh lemon juice
1 pint of sour cream
3 tablespoons of flour
1 cup of brown sugar
3 tablespoons cornstarch
4 large eggs

1. Preheat oven to 325 degrees and slide a pan of water on the lower rack of the oven.
2. Mix together cream cheese, ricotta and sour cream. Fold in the brown sugar and mix in remaining ingredients (except the pomegranate arils) one at a time and mix everything thoroughly.
3. Pour the mixture into a greased 9-inch spring form pan and place pan on the middle rack of the oven on 350 degrees for 1 hour. Once

that hour is up, turn the oven off, but leave the cheesecake in the oven for an additional hour.

4. Let the cheesecake cool on a wire rack. Refrigerate overnight.
5. When it is time to serve the cheesecake, cover the top completely in pomegranate arils. Cut and serve.

****** And now... a little something just for Mom and Dad ******

POMEGRANATE DIRTY MARTINI

1 bottle of pomegranate twist mix (most grocery beverage store sells them)
1 bottle of olive juice
1 Grey Goose Vodka bottle
1 jar of green olives
Ice cubes

1. Fill the shaker 1/4 with ice cubes
2. Pour in 2oz vodka, 5oz pomegranate martini mix and 1.5oz olive juice
3. Replace the cap. Shake well
4. Pour your fabulous mixed drink into martini glasses and garnish with olive

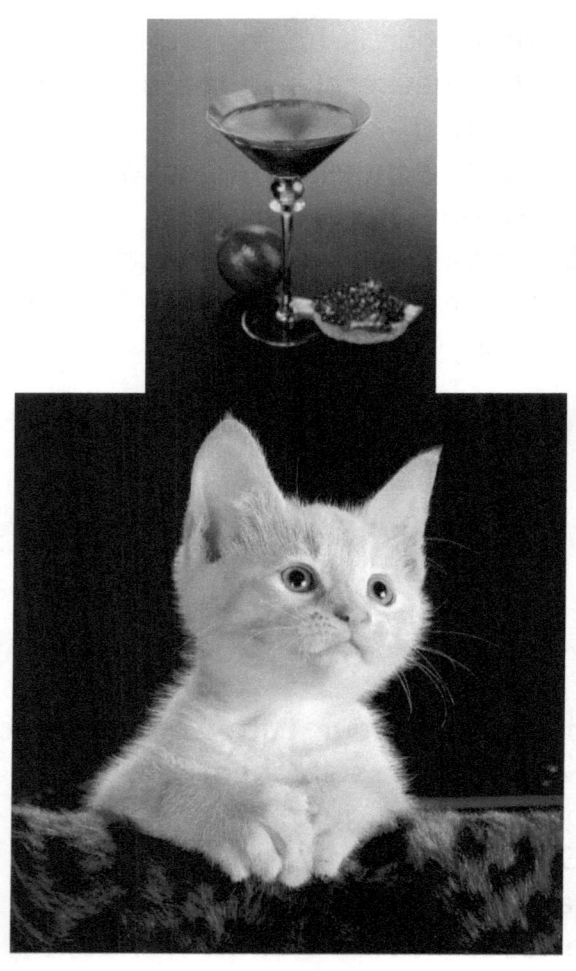

If you like my book, Please give me a review, I sure would appreciate your help. Thank you soooo much!!!!!!!!!

REFERENCES

Adi. (2012, July 18). *Pomegranate – Medicinal Uses & Ayurvedic Home Remedies.* Retrieved from Indiatva: http://www.indiatva.com/pomegranate-medicinal-uses-ayurvedic-home-remedies

Aviram, M., Dornfield, L., Rosenblat, M., Volkova, N., Kaplan, M., Coleman, R., & Fuhrman, B. (2000). Pomegranate juice consumption reduces oxidative stress, atherogenic modifications to LDL, and platelet aggregation: studies in humans and in atherosclerotic apolipoprotein E–deficient mice. *The American Journal of Clinical Nutrition*, 1062-1076.

Aviram, M., Rosenblat, M., Gaitini, D., Nitecki, S., Hoffman, A., Dornfield, A., & Hayek, T. (2004). Pomegranate juice consumption for 3 years by patients with carotid artery stenosis reduces common carotid intima-media thickness, blood pressure and LDL oxidation. *Clinical Nutrition*, 423-433.

Barnes, L. (n.d.). *Pomegranate.* Retrieved from Plantdex: http://www.plantdex.com/index.php/species-growing-guides/fruits/129-pomegranate

Barnes, L. (n.d.). *Varieties of Pomegranate Trees.* Retrieved from Plantdex: http://www.plantdex.com/index.php/plant-pulp-monthly/289-varities-of-pomegranate-trees

Bowden, J. (n.d.). *The 10 Best Foods You Aren't Eating.* Retrieved from Men's Health: http://www.menshealth.com/mhlists/best_healthy_foods/Pomegranate_Juice.php

Christman, S. (2003, September 3). *Punica Granatum.* Retrieved from Floridata: http://www.floridata.com/ref/P/puni_gra.cfm

Daniells, S. (2006, March 6). *Pomegranate Peel Extract Has 'More Potential' as Supplement.* Retrieved from Nutra Ingredients: http://www.nutraingredients.com/Research/Pomegranate-peel-extract-has-more-potential-as-supplement

Derrick, D. (2011). *Fruit of the Month - Pomegranate.* Retrieved from KDD: http://www.kddc.com/fruitsofmonth.aspx

FAQ: Everything You Wanted to Know About Pomegranates. (n.d.). Retrieved from Pomegranates: http://pomegranates.org/index.php?c=7

Find a Vitamin or Supplement: Pomegranate. (n.d.). Retrieved from WebMD: http://www.webmd.com/vitamins-supplements/ingredientmono-392-

POMEGRANATE.aspx?activeIngredientId=392&activeIngredientName=POM EGRANATE

Fortini, A. (2008, March 31). *Pomegranate Princess*. Retrieved from The New Yorker: http://www.newyorker.com/reporting/2008/03/31/080331fa_fact_fortini

How many seeds does a pomegranate have? (n.d.). Retrieved from Aqua Phoenix: http://www.aquaphoenix.com/misc/pomegranate/

Jackson-Michel, S. (2010, November 17). *Pomegranate Seed Oil Benefits*. Retrieved from LiveStrong: http://www.livestrong.com/article/310383-pomegranate-seed-oil-benefits/

Mandal, A. (n.d.). *What are Antioxidants?* Retrieved from News Medical: http://www.news-medical.net/health/What-are-Antioxidants.aspx

Melendez, L. (n.d.). *What Are Pomegranates Good For?* Retrieved from EHow: http://www.ehow.com/about_5422683_pomegranates-good.html#page=0

Patisaul, H., & Jefferson, W. (2010, March 27). *The Pros and Cons of Phytoestrogens*. Retrieved from US National Library of Medicine Nationa Institutes of Health: http://www.ncbi.nlm.nih.gov/pmc/articles/PMC3074428/

Pomegranate. (n.d.). Retrieved from Herb Wisdom: http://www.herbwisdom.com/herb-pomegranates.html

Pomegranate. (n.d.). Retrieved from http://www.hort.purdue.edu/newcrop/morton/pomegranate.html

Pomegranate. (n.d.). Retrieved from http://www.crfg.org/pubs/ff/pomegranate.html

Pomegranate. (2012, January 1). Retrieved from University of Maryland Medical Center: http://umm.edu/health/medical/altmed/herb/pomegranate

Pomegranate Juice, Bottled. (n.d.). Retrieved from Agricultural Research Service United States Department of Agriculture: http://ndb.nal.usda.gov/ndb/foods/show/2516?fg=&man=&lfacet=&format=&count=&max=25&offset=&sort=&qlookup=pomegranate

Pomegranate Nutrition Facts. (n.d.). Retrieved from Nutrition and You: http://www.nutrition-and-you.com/pomegranate.html

Pomegranate Seed Oil. (n.d.). Retrieved from I Love India: http://www.iloveindia.com/indian-herbs/pomegranate-seed-oil.html

Pomegranates, Raw. (n.d.). Retrieved from Nutrition Data: http://nutritiondata.self.com/facts/fruits-and-fruit-juices/2038/2

Pomegranates, Raw. (n.d.). Retrieved from Agricultural Research Service United States Department of Agriculture: http://ndb.nal.usda.gov/ndb/foods/show/2434?fg=&man=&lfacet=&format=&count=&max=25&offset=&sort=&qlookup=pomegranate

Romero, M. (2012, May 17). *Why Pomegranate Seeds are Good for You*. Retrieved from Washingtonian: http://www.washingtonian.com/blogs/wellbeing/nutrition/why-pomegranate-seeds-are-so-good-for-you.php

Shipman, M. (2013, September 19). *Pomegranate Export Markets Growing*. Retrieved from The Packer: http://www.thepacker.com/fruit-vegetable-news/Pomegranate-export-markets-growing-224449751.html

Striepe, B. (2012, August 12). *Superfood: 10 Delicious Pomegranate Recipes*. Retrieved from Care 2 : http://www.care2.com/greenliving/superfood-pomegranate-health-benefits-tips.html

Vrouvas, M. (n.d.). *What Are the Dangers of Pomegranate Juice*. Retrieved from EHow Health: http://www.ehow.com/facts_5519835_dangers-pomegranate-juice.html

What is Pomegranate Seed Oil? (n.d.). Retrieved from Wise Geek: http://www.wisegeek.com/what-is-pomegranate-seed-oil.htm

Who needs Viagra? The secret to enhancing your sex drive could be a daily glass of pomegranate juice. (2012, May 4). Retrieved from Mirror: http://www.mirror.co.uk/news/technology-science/science/is-pomegranate-juice-the-new-viagra-study-817875

Wolf, B. (2006, November 1). *Pomegranates: Jewels in the Fruit Crown*. Retrieved from NPR: http://www.npr.org/2011/07/15/6411097/pomegranates-jewels-in-the-fruit-crown

IMAGES

An opened up pomegranate by SriniG on August 6, 2006
Image source: http://en.wikipedia.org/wiki/File:Pomegranate_opened.jpg

Pomegranate by കാക്കര
Image source: http://commons.wikimedia.org/wiki/File:Pomegranate_-
_%E0%B4%AE%E0%B4%BE%E0%B4%A4%E0%B4%B3%E0%B4%A8%E0%B4%B
E%E0%B4%B0%E0%B4%95%E0%B4%82_02.JPG

Pomegranate seeds by Stacy Spensley on November 19, 2010
Image source: http://www.flickr.com/photos/notahipster/5190365991/

Pomegranate tree by Four Years on October 17, 2008
Image source: http://www.flickr.com/photos/2009seasons/4098005173/

Pomegranate by fir0002 / Lucas on July 12, 2012
Image source: http://www.flickr.com/photos/ancientartpodcast/8045324905/

Pomegranate 2 by Lelivingandco at http://lelivingandco.blogspot.ca on October 30,
2012
Image source: http://www.flickr.com/photos/lelivingandco/8143287513/

India - Koyambedu Market - Pomegranate 01 by McKaySavage on October 5, 2009
Image source: http://www.fotopedia.com/items/flickr-3986294387

Soak the Pomegranate by Mat Honan
Image source: http://www.flickr.com/photos/honan/1665551847/in/set-
72157602572977955/

Step Five Break the Fruit Apart by Mat Honan
Image source: http://www.flickr.com/photos/honan/1666411094/

Pomegranate Seeds by Michelle Tribe / Greencollander on September 27, 2008
Image source: http://www.flickr.com/photos/greencolander/2895452690/

Pomegranate Seeds, Macro -1 by Zeeweez on January 16, 2012
Image source: http://www.flickr.com/photos/zeevveez/6706587433/

Pomegranates at Casa de Mari by Mari Smith on October 10, 2010
Image source:
http://www.flickr.com/photos/marismith/5069353254/sizes/m/in/photolist-
8HXL7j-aTcdvH-4RsE9R-6vA26V-64bRXD-4DA4P4-4DEmfo-7dDyC4-fnoJ6g-fnCWsu-
64bMYk-dEjfdg-2Ve3dn-fcSjgR-7f8ogM-7QkqX3-7f8oTr-ag83as-54o5UU-7f8maB-
7fceRN-bgix4k-3jXTP6-5TvyFi-7efPCG-8LdjUh-7ytdpf-7dHnKL-8j6HE8-cTWSj5-

7dDwzD-bypKKa-7agfTG-2XBt9s-4RsE1x-a6RMMo-c2Xa5L-7V8KbK-fbmHHQ-9htEyk-7tdXCF-6VPJRo-2vZBsG-7thVpE-9Naa8N-4U3YCH-6Ls2LF-6n2Gke-6n2GiD-6n6S2N-5sZRDq/

Pomegranate Arils by w:User:Pschemp on December 21, 2005
Image source: http://en.wikipedia.org/wiki/File:Pomseeds2.jpg

English Farmer / Anar (Pomegranate) by Bhanji11 on January 11, 2013
Image source:
http://commons.wikimedia.org/wiki/File:Anar%28Pomegranate%29.jpg

Kisir with a Twist I by Blue Moon in Her Eyes on October 21, 2010
Image source:
http://www.flickr.com/photos/bluumwezi/5102154031/sizes/m/in/photolist-8LRSCX-8LRSU2-3xbiHx-wJHHi-dbpz2X-ekUrmU-7KeMSj-8Jd7Zb-2zQJMV-67Cz3a-ayV9Nm-5EvtkU-5Erbic-5Erbvr-5EreHT-5Evu8E-5ErdQV-5EvtqU-5Erbop/

Lemon Myrtile Essential Oil in Clear Glass Vile by ItinerantTrader on February 22, 2009
Image source: http://en.wikipedia.org/wiki/File:LemonMyrtleEssentialOil.png

Feet on Scale by Bill Branson
Image source: https://en.m.wikipedia.org/wiki/File:Feet_on_scale.jpg

Pomegranate Series by Thor / Geishaboy500
Image source:
http://www.flickr.com/photos/49503154413@N01/3047089636/in/photolist-5Dg8Ad-bazjRa-51gHJq-5DbPDZ-cUpeoL-aaN7SN-do6frS-do6fx7-do67Ce-fMwV4g-4gGQPg-4CDgBx-vryd9-6Nevcm-8jGcYi-yYTmu-dWDHbh-7mcdsj-7mcdDs-7mcdR1-7m8kRa-7m8jZv-neAQA-5NvLA8-6aTdqX-9YEa1Z-5dZSbn-7Knp5h-7KisTR-9ciES-2tNJ1J-Dc91g-e7RLjh-7PKT1G-ez6Eas-9BcfTC-bP41Fx-9bimWx-67UiMZ-5vpbRH-4ibzDZ-9DaoqR-4ifEoA-8WcDVa-7L5dLR-2RCfZt-8yGqNr-6ovP4L-88y1f-cZmUYs-5jA4fV

Pomegranate Molasses by Jules Morgan on November 7, 2009
Image source: http://www.flickr.com/photos/ladymissmarquise/6252346449/

Crepes by Kimberly Vardeman on February 8, 2009
Image source:
http://www.flickr.com/photos/kimberlykv/3265498052/sizes/m/in/photolist-5YywNy-9jd3EB-ouZxH-5YyFaC-7DYur9-7a9jDF-6MchRG-6Vxdc2-7nuVVk-6nSW9E-btyZMB-fcLbrn-5ANFBa-ejC6tt-3Z7mPQ-5GSTbu-7n481c-ejHSFf-f6VEyf-5WxM57-5Wtvd8-85DZvK-64Dsic-5VEeFV-7GdpnU-u1Nmk-u1Nik-6RpaoA-6AoZro-4Pogmt-rM5rR-cQxLnh-5YyvKb-5Yyxkm-5XB9Z1-7esbNZ-8gRWus-9ofejF-5BQk29-5YyAW1-5YyEqs-5YyCgN-5YupAD-5ZvPzW-5Yyzpu-5bBE37-7DUELa-bB5Ryx-7DUEPX-7DYuXC-t3kXn/

IMG_5107 by Neeta Lind on March 17, 2011
Image source:
http://www.flickr.com/photos/71132408@N00/5538996282/in/photolist-9rsNBU-7v27Fe-7v5Wd3-5PJvF9-4DLs6s-54y5Qs-4LcbYv

Hibiscus by Joey / Joo0ey on July 30, 2011
Image source:
http://www.flickr.com/photos/joo0ey/5996109796/sizes/m/in/photolist-a8RCxo-5VwtSV-73eWTa-acAunH-4Uc6bh-acAunt-9nGSG7-7Beu4d-7oHtvh-9MJXi6-7tLf66-fQfFQ-xK7CA-9DGRoG-fc82Zn-bRJhYk-fLpPYg-aqTCdL-9QZ4Qq-63A5NT-8cPrRH-8cPpER-ck6uNu-7td4K2-73iVzS-7BQJQY-7BQJSy-7UTUSL-82cvPw-94b7cA-8XW6GW-7BaEbM-7Beu29-7oDAJB-38Bwr1-bCsZeo-wEAWB-MBFA5-biCH3e-4LtCQF-bK2tA4-eJnm5y-eJnm53-eJggLP-eJghkV-eJggMT-eJggLe-eJnm7w-eJnm93-eJnm4q-eJggPX/